MILITARY WORKOUT

Train Like a Soldier: The Complete Military Workout Plan for Strength, Fat Loss, and Mental Toughness

ZERO EXCUSES PUBLISHING

Table of Contents

1. Why Train Like a Soldier

What separates a soldier from an average person isn't just strength or stamina — it's mindset. It's the ability to keep going when the body says stop. It's the discipline to wake up and show up, whether it's raining, freezing, or you just don't feel like it. That's what this book is about: not just transforming your body, but forging the mental toughness that lasts long after the workout is over.

You're holding a practical, no-excuses guide to military-style fitness. This is not a theory book. It's a mission-ready program built to deliver results using your bodyweight, minimal equipment, and maximum effort. Whether you're just getting started or returning to serious training, this plan meets you where you are — and demands you move forward.

Military training doesn't rely on fads, gimmicks, or fancy machines. It's based on raw, proven methods designed to build strong, lean, capable bodies in the toughest environments. In this book, you'll find everything you need to train like a soldier — no matter your current level.

Here's what you can expect:

- **Clarity** – You'll know exactly what to do, how to do it, and when. No fluff, no confusion.

- **Progression** – Whether you're a beginner or advanced, you'll find a path that pushes you without overwhelming you.

- **Mental Edge** – Each chapter strengthens more than your body. You'll build focus, resilience, and self-discipline.

- **Real Results** – Strength, fat loss, endurance, and confidence — if you put in the work.

This program is divided into clear, progressive phases. You'll begin by building the mindset and setting your mission goals. From there, you'll move into the core training plans — a 6-week tactical program, optional fat-loss and strength tracks, and practical nutrition strategies that fuel performance. We'll also cover how to recover smarter, avoid injury, and keep improving long after the first six weeks are over.

You don't need perfect conditions. You don't need to "feel ready." You just need to start.

If you want flashy workouts with zero substance, this isn't your book. If you're looking for a system that sharpens both your body and your mind — welcome to the mission.

Let's begin.

2. The Soldier's Mindset

Before the first push-up.
Before the first drop of sweat.
Before the first day of training, comes mindset.

In the military, your mind is your first and most important weapon. Physical strength means nothing if the mind gives up when things get hard. That's why soldiers are trained to think differently, long before they ever step onto the field. And if you want to train like a soldier, you have to adopt the same mindset.

Discipline Over Motivation

Forget motivation. It's a fair-weather friend — here one day, gone the next. It shows up when you're excited, but then disappears when the work gets hard.

Discipline is the friend that remains. When the motivation is gone, when you feel tired, or you forget your goal, discipline is there for you.

Soldiers don't rely on motivation to get through 5 a.m. runs, long ruck marches, or cold training nights. They rely on habit. Routine. Purpose. They show up because it's their duty — and that's the mindset you'll need for this program. You won't always want to train. That's fine, that's even normal. But you must do it anyway: the only way to be disciplined is to never give up.

The discipline you're about to build here won't just get you in shape (the body is just a piece of a puzzle: *mens sana in corpore sano*) – this discipline will carry over to everything else in life.

Routine Builds Results

In military life, routine isn't boring — it's powerful. Repeating small actions with intention builds mastery. Showing up day after day — even when the progress feels slow — is how real results are made.

That's why this program is structured around clear, consistent action: daily workouts, simple goals, repeatable habits. You'll know what to do and when to do it. It's your job to execute.

Stick to the routine. Trust the process. The results will come.

Mental Toughness = Controlled Response Under Stress

Mental toughness isn't about being emotionless or aggressive. It's about staying calm, focused, and effective under pressure — when your body is tired, when life gets in the way, when nothing is going according to plan.

Every workout you push through builds this toughness. Every skipped excuse makes you stronger. And the more you train, the more you'll learn: discomfort is exactly where you grow. Embrace it.

Accountability Is a Personal Responsibility

In the military, you're responsible for your gear, your team, your time, and your results. No one is coming to save you — and no one can do the reps for you. That same personal accountability applies here.

If you miss a day, own it. If you fall off track, reset and keep moving. No guilt. No excuses. Just action.

Track your workouts. Set goals. Write things down. Hold yourself to a standard.

You're not just "trying to get in shape" — you're building a new standard for yourself.

Progress, Not Perfection: Done is better than perfect

This program isn't about being perfect on day 1. It's about being better than you were yesterday. Progress comes in inches, not miles. What really matters is momentum. You don't have to train like a Navy SEAL from day one. You just have to train. With each rep, each workout, each week — you level up.

The soldier's mindset isn't about hype. It's about quiet consistency, earned confidence, and showing up regardless of how you feel that day.

You're not here to talk about it.
You're here to do the work.
Now let's move.

3. The Mission: Set Your Fitness Objectives

Train with clarity, purpose, and results.

In the military, you don't wake up and "see how it goes." You wake up with orders. You have a mission. You execute.

That's the mindset you need to bring into your training. If you're just "trying to get in shape," your results will be inconsistent, and your motivation will fade. But if you train with purpose — with clear, measurable objectives — your discipline becomes sharper, your progress becomes visible, and your workouts become something more than physical. They become part of your mission.

This chapter is about choosing your fitness objective, understanding how your body adapts to training, and setting up a 6-week plan with precision.

Why Vague Goals Don't Work

Too many people make goals like:

- "I just want to lose weight."
- "I want to look better."
- "I want to be fitter."

That's not a mission. That's a mood.

A mission is clear. It's measurable. It has deadlines. In a real military context, a vague order can cost lives. In fitness, it costs you time, energy, and results.

You don't need a perfect plan. You need a specific one. The more clearly you define your mission, the more likely you are to execute it — even when motivation fades.

The 3 Core Mission Types

Most people fall into one of three categories. Some combine them, but it helps to pick one as your **primary** focus so your training and mindset stay locked in.

1. Fat Loss

Your mission: reduce body fat while maintaining muscle.

What it requires:

- High-effort training (circuits, intervals, conditioning)
- Clean, structured nutrition (caloric deficit, high protein)
- Daily movement, hydration, and recovery

What to track:

- Waist and hip circumference
- Progress photos (every 2 weeks)
- How clothes fit
- Scale weight (optional — but don't obsess over it)

Mental tip: Fat loss happens when you stay consistent, not when you starve. The mission is sustainability — not short-term suffering.

2. Strength

Your mission: increase muscular control, power, and ability to perform more reps or harder movements.

What it requires:

- Progressive overload: more reps, harder variations, shorter rest
- Solid form and full range of motion
- Focus on core compound movements (push-ups, pull-ups, squats, planks, dips, etc.)

What to track:

- Max push-ups in 2 minutes
- Pull-ups without assistance
- Controlled reps of squats, dips, planks, lunges
- Quality over quantity

Mental tip: Strength isn't just about brute force — it's control under tension. Your body learns what you repeatedly demand of it.

3. Endurance

Your mission: improve stamina, recovery speed, and physical performance under stress.

What it requires:

- Cardio-based circuits
- Longer, steady-state runs and/or rucks
- Breathing control and pacing
- Building fatigue resistance over time

What to track:

- Time to complete circuits
- 1.5-mile and 2-mile run times
- Recovery heart rate
- Duration of continuous effort

Always keep in mind that <u>endurance is mental before it's physical</u>. Your lungs will scream — your mind must decide whether to quit or continue.

Training Adaptation: The Science Behind Improvement

To set effective goals, you need to understand how progress actually happens.

Your body adapts to what it's exposed to. The process is known as the SAID Principle, which stands for *Specific Adaptation to Imposed Demands.*

That means:

- If you lift heavy → your body builds strength
- If you run often → your body improves oxygen efficiency
- If you do high-rep circuits → your endurance improves
- If you do nothing → your body adapts to rest

Training is a conversation with your body. What you say (through workouts), it responds to.

But this only works if three things are present:

1. **Progressive overload** – You challenge yourself more over time
2. **Recovery** – You rest and fuel adequately
3. **Consistency** – You train regularly, not randomly

Set a Clear 6-Week Objective

This program is structured around a 6-week cycle — short enough to maintain focus, long enough to make visible change.

Let's walk through building your personal training mission.

➤ 1. Establish Your Starting Point

Take 20 minutes to:

- Perform the **assessment workouts** in Chapter 4
- Measure your waist, hips, chest, arms
- Take front and side photos
- Write down how you feel physically and mentally

This is your "Day 0." You'll look back at this in 6 weeks and see just how far you've come.

➤ 2. Write a **SMART** Goal

SMART goals are such a simple yet effective concept: sometimes simplicity is key. Setting some impossible or unsustainable goals might be even worse than having no goals at all. When we set an unrealistic goal, we try our best for a few days before giving up, and when this happens, we create a certain negative pattern that will negatively affect us in the future.

SMART goals have a few characteristics:

- **S**pecific – "Lose 2 kg" not "get lean"

- **M**easurable – You can track it

- **A**chievable – 5 kg fat loss in 6 weeks? Maybe. 15 kg? Not safely.

- **R**ealistic – You have a life. Be honest.

- **T**ime-bound – This program = 6 weeks. That's your deadline.

Let's see some examples to better understand what I mean:

- "Lose 4 cm from my waist and do 20 push-ups without stopping."

- "Improve my 2-mile run time from 18 minutes to 15:30."

- "Complete every workout in the 6-week plan without missing a day."

Write your goal now. Don't skip this. When the work gets hard, this is what pulls you through.

➤ 3. Plan Your Weekly Check-ins

Every Sunday, take at least 10 minutes to:

- Log your performance (reps, time, weight) – how did the week go? What can you improve? What are you proud of?

- Reflect on your energy, consistency, and mood

- Adjust your food, sleep, or pacing if needed – test/find concrete solutions to boost your energy levels and improve

Use the **training journal in the appendix** to track it all. You don't need perfection. You need momentum.

A 1% improvement every week leads to a massive change in just 6 weeks.

➤ 4. Visualize the Finish Line

Close your eyes. Picture yourself in 6 weeks:

- How does your body feel?
- What can you do now that you couldn't before?
- How do your clothes fit?
- What does your confidence feel like?

This is more than a workout plan. This is a personal transformation mission. And every mission begins with a vision.

Accountability: Be Your Own Commander

You don't need a coach yelling in your ear. You need personal responsibility. That's what this training builds — and that's why it works.

No one is watching. No one is grading your reps. But you are either executing or making excuses.

You don't have to be perfect — but you do have to be honest. Did you show up? Did you try? Did you stick to the plan even when it got hard?

Progress is built in the moment when you could quit — but choose not to.

Final Orders

Your mission is set when:

- You know your primary goal
- You understand how your body adapts
- You've chosen your target and timeline
- You're ready to execute

Next, we move into **the physical foundations** — how military workouts are structured, what makes them different, and how you'll train for real-world strength, stamina, and resilience.

Gear up. The mission has begun.

4. Military Fitness Basics

Before you jump into push-ups, sprints, and circuits, you need to understand how this training works, and more importantly, why it works. Military training isn't magic. It's not trendy. It's not built around flashy gear, social media aesthetics, or gym theatrics. It's designed to prepare a person to function under pressure — physically, mentally, and emotionally — using simple, proven methods that build real-world capability.

This chapter lays out the fundamentals behind military-style fitness. These are the principles that shape every workout in the pages ahead — principles that don't just make you sweat, but make you ready. If you want to train like a soldier, you have to understand how a soldier trains.

Fitness that Serves a Purpose

In the civilian world, fitness is often framed as a form of self-image. People work out to look a certain way, to hit a number on the scale, or to chase some vague idea of "healthy." While there's nothing wrong with wanting to feel confident in your own body, military fitness doesn't stop at surface-level goals.

For soldiers, training is about function first. A soldier trains so they can climb, crawl, run, carry, pull, and fight. Aesthetics are irrelevant if you can't perform under stress. And more often than not, the result of this functional focus is a strong, lean, durable body — not because that's the goal, but because it's the consequence of training for real ability.

This program follows the same path. We're not sculpting bodies for the beach. We're building them for battle — and in doing so, you'll create something far more satisfying than just "looking good." You'll create a body that can perform.

Efficiency Over Complexity

The beauty of military training is its simplicity. While the fitness industry constantly tries to reinvent itself with new gadgets and complicated routines, military fitness sticks to the basics. It relies on movements that have stood the test of time — push-ups, pull-ups, squats, rucking, running, core control — and applies them consistently, with increasing intensity.

This program doesn't require fancy equipment or specialized machines. Most of the work will be done using your own bodyweight, a floor, and some basic gear if you have it (a backpack, a pull-up bar, maybe a sandbag). Why? These are the tools that soldiers use in the field.

They're accessible. They're scalable. And they force your body to work as one coordinated system, not a collection of disconnected muscle groups.

This kind of efficiency is what makes the training portable — you can do it at home, outdoors, or even in a small apartment. There are no excuses, because there are no barriers.

Total Body Integration

A common mistake in modern training is thinking of the body in pieces — a "chest day," a "leg day," an "arm day." But in combat or emergencies, your body doesn't act in isolated segments. It acts as a unit.

When you're sprinting toward cover, dragging a partner to safety, or lifting your pack overhead, you're using your entire system — muscles, joints, lungs, heart, and nervous system — all working together.

Military fitness emphasizes total-body movement. That's why you'll find exercises in this program that demand coordination, balance, core stability, and stamina at the same time. A simple movement like a push-up isn't just an arm exercise — it trains your chest, shoulders, triceps, core, and mental focus. A loaded ruck march isn't just about your legs — it works your back, grip, posture, and discipline.

When your training treats the body like a system — instead of isolated parts — you build real-life readiness. The strength you gain becomes useful strength. The stamina you build becomes usable stamina. It transfers from the training floor to your everyday world.

Bodyweight Doesn't Mean Easy

Let's kill a myth right now: bodyweight training is not "beginner" training. In fact, some of the most challenging, high-level fitness work you can do requires nothing more than your own body — and gravity.

Ask any Marine, SEAL, or special operator how many push-ups or pull-ups they've done in their life. You won't hear them talk about bench press maxes. You'll hear about how many rounds they can last, how long they can hang, how fast they can move with 30 pounds on their back.

That's the kind of training we're doing here.

Bodyweight training develops strength-to-weight ratio — your ability to move and control your own body. It's not just about lifting — it's about handling. Think of it like this: if you can't control your own body with precision, you're not ready to carry more.

The advantage of bodyweight work is its scalability. A push-up can be made easier by elevating the hands, or harder by changing the tempo or angle. A squat can be loaded with a ruck or made explosive with a jump.

You're always progressing — but never relying on a machine to move the weight for you.

Cardio Is More Than Running

Conditioning is often misunderstood. People associate it with long, boring runs — but in a military setting, cardio has range. It includes interval sprints, circuits, rucking, and tactical endurance drills that challenge your heart, lungs, legs, and willpower all at once.

In this program, you won't be logging endless miles unless your goal demands it. Instead, we focus on mission-style cardio: running with purpose, moving with urgency, and training in ways that improve oxygen efficiency, recovery speed, and mental toughness.

You'll sweat, yes. But more importantly, you'll build the kind of durable engine that keeps going when others stop.

Core: The Unsung Hero

Every military movement — running, crawling, climbing, lifting, throwing — requires a strong, stable core. And yet, most people treat core training like an afterthought. A few crunches at the end of a session and they're done.

This book takes a different approach. Core training is not about doing 100 sit-ups. It's about building the deep internal control that protects your spine, supports your posture, and links your upper and lower body together under stress.

That's why you'll be training the core with holds, carries, dynamic movement, and bracing drills — the kind that soldiers rely on when moving under load.

And instead of chasing burn, you'll chase function. Because a functional core doesn't just look good — it performs.

Mobility: The Shield That Keeps You Moving

Mobility isn't glamorous, but it's essential. Soldiers train to move well in unpredictable conditions — over uneven terrain, through tight spaces, under load. If your joints don't move freely, or your muscles are tight and unbalanced, your risk of injury skyrockets.

That's why this program includes mobility and flexibility work — not as a warm-up side note, but as an essential part of your weekly routine. You'll learn how to loosen up tight hips and shoulders, how to open your thoracic spine for better breathing and posture, and how to maintain range of motion in your ankles, knees, and wrists — all without hours of stretching.

A few smart, intentional drills will keep you in the game longer and performing at a higher level.

What This Chapter Is (and Isn't)

This chapter isn't here to give you a science textbook. You don't need to memorize muscle fiber types or energy system charts. You need to understand the basics of what you're about to do, why it works, and how to approach it like a professional — even if you're just starting out.

Here's the reality: this program works because it uses the same approach applied to tens of thousands of military trainees every year. It strips away the non-essentials, focuses on what delivers results, and demands consistency. That's it.

There are no hacks. No shortcuts. But also no confusion. You're not here to be busy — you're here to be better. And the only way to get better is to master the basics, show up, and execute. Again and again.

5. Preparing for Battle: Assessments & Readiness

Before any operation, soldiers run through checks: equipment, readiness, terrain, and mission brief. This chapter is your personal pre-mission checklist. No hype, no guesswork. Just the data and protocols you need to find your baseline and prepare your body to train effectively and safely.

You'll complete:

- A functional fitness test based on military benchmarks
- A mobility screening to spot movement limitations
- A mental readiness scan
- An injury-prevention overview
- A simple warm-up routine to use before every workout

You can't improve what you don't measure. This isn't about comparing yourself to others — it's about identifying where you are right now so you can choose the right level of training intensity and track real progress.

Treat this like recon. You're gathering intel to execute the mission better.

Step 1: The Tactical Fitness Assessment

This test measures functional performance — not gym numbers or aesthetics. It's inspired by the U.S. Army Combat Fitness Test (ACFT), Navy Physical Readiness Test (PRT), and elements of the Marine PFT. You'll perform these in sequence with rest between efforts.

Record your reps, time, and form. Keep it honest.

Test   **Protocol:**
Rest 2–3 minutes between exercises. Warm up beforehand (use the warm-up later in this chapter).

1. **Push-Ups – Max in 2 Minutes**
   - o Chest must lower to at least a closed fist's height from the ground.
   - o Elbows lock out at the top.
   - o Modified version: on knees (beginner)

2. **Sit-Ups – Max in 2 Minutes**
   - o Feet anchored or flat, knees bent.
   - o Hands behind ears or crossed over chest (don't pull your neck).
   - o Shoulder blades must touch ground on each rep.

3. **Bodyweight Squats – Max in 2 Minutes**
   - o Hip crease below knees at bottom.
   - o Heels flat, chest up.
   - o Count only clean reps.

4. **1.5-Mile Run – Timed**
   - o Standard distance for military conditioning.
   - o Run, jog, or run-walk — but keep moving.
   - o Mark your time and note your breathing, pacing, and recovery.

Optional Add-Ons (if you want more data):

- **Plank Hold for Time** (Target: 1+ minute)
- **Pull-Ups or Inverted Rows – Max Reps**
- **Burpees – Max in 1 Minute**

Scoring   &   Interpreting   Your   Results
This isn't about ranking. It's about level-setting. Use the ranges below to get a sense of your current fitness status:

Test	Beginner	Intermediate	Advanced
Push-Ups (2min)	<15	15–35	35+
Sit-Ups (2min)	<20	20–45	45+
Squats (2 min)	<30	30–60	60+
1.5-Mile Run	14+ min	11:30–14 min	<11:30

Assignment:

Write your numbers down. You'll compare them again after the 6-week program. If you're in the Beginner range on most tests, start with the basic plan. If you're Intermediate or Advanced, you'll have progression tracks in the training phase. Either way — you're not stuck. Every score here can and will improve with work

.

Step 2: Mobility & Movement Screening

Before loading the system, check the joints. Limited mobility means limited performance — and higher injury risk.

Here's a basic diagnostic you can do at home in 5–10 minutes.

Mobility Checklist:

1. **Deep Squat Test**
   o   Stand with feet shoulder-width.
   o   Squat as deep as possible while keeping heels flat.
   o   Can you get your hips below your knees without rounding your back or lifting heels?
   o   If not: work on hip and ankle mobility.

2. **Overhead Reach Test**
   o   Stand tall, feet together.
   o   Reach both arms overhead with palms facing in.
   o   Can you get your biceps in line with your ears without arching your lower back?

o If not: shoulder or thoracic (upper back) mobility is
limited.

3. **Straight Leg Raise**

   o Lie flat on your back.

   o Raise one leg while keeping the other flat on the floor.

   o Can you raise to about 80–90 degrees (straight leg, no
   bent knee)?

   o If not: tight hamstrings or hip flexors.

4. **Wrist Extension Test**

   o Place palms flat on the floor in front of you with
   fingers forward.

   o Can your shoulders pass directly over your hands
   without pain?

   o If not: limited wrist or forearm flexibility.

Assignment:

Note any movements that feel tight, restricted, or painful. These don't
disqualify you from training — they just signal that your warm-ups
should include targeted mobility drills. We'll include these later on in
the plan.

Step 3: Mental Readiness Brief

This isn't a motivational pep talk. It's a short reality check.

Training success is about consistency, and consistency is often
blocked by poor planning — not poor effort.

Ask yourself:

• Can I commit 30–45 minutes a day, 4–6 days a week, for the
next 6 weeks?

• Do I have space to train (home, gym, outdoors)?

• Am I willing to follow one program without constantly
switching?

• Can I log my progress weekly?

- Do I have basic nutrition under control (or am I ready to improve it)?

If you answered "no" to any of these, it's not a failure. It's nothing but a warning sign. Adapt your plan to reality. Maybe start with 3 days a week and build up. Maybe train in the morning before distractions hit. But be honest: if your setup isn't ready, neither are your results. Don't be afraid of your results, don't be afraid of your reality: discipline and time will adjust reality to your goals. Remember that it's not

Step 4: Injury Prevention Essentials

The best way to stay consistent is to stay healthy.

Here's what you need to know:

- **Warm-Up Properly:** Don't skip this. A rushed body is a vulnerable body.

- **Train with Form First:** No sloppy reps. Clean movement builds real strength.

- **Don't Ignore Pain:** Soreness is normal. Sharp pain is not.

- **Sleep Matters:** Recovery = gains. Under-slept = underperforming.

- **Hydrate + Fuel:** A dehydrated soldier is a slower, weaker soldier.

You don't need a sports medicine degree. You need common sense and body awareness. If something doesn't feel right — scale back, modify, or rest.

Step 5: The Standard Warm-Up Protocol

Use this before every training session. It preps your muscles, joints, nervous system, and mind for effort.

Dynamic Warm-Up – 5 to 8 Minutes

1. Arm Circles – 30 seconds each direction
2. Leg Swings (front-to-back + side-to-side) – 10 each leg
3. Hip Circles – 10 each direction

4. World's Greatest Stretch – 3 reps each side

5. Inchworm Walkouts – 5 reps

6. Bodyweight Squats – 10 reps

7. Jumping Jacks – 30 seconds

8. Light Jog in Place or Shadowboxing – 30 seconds

That's it. Simple. Efficient. Effective.

6. The 6-Week Tactical Fitness Plan

You've built the mindset.

You've set your mission.

You've learned the principles behind military training.

Now it's time to execute.

This is the heart of the book — a 6-week tactical training plan built on real-world principles. It's designed to challenge your body, sharpen your discipline, and create noticeable progress. You won't need a gym. You won't need machines. Just your body, a pull-up bar or backpack (if available), and the willingness to push yourself further than yesterday.

This plan is progressive, structured, and adaptable. Whether you're a beginner just starting out or an experienced athlete looking to reset and rebuild, this chapter gives you the tools to train like a soldier — with purpose and precision.

How the Program Works

The training is divided into six weeks, each building on the last. You'll train five days per week, with two dedicated rest or recovery days. Each day has a clear purpose:

- **Day 1: Strength + Core**
- **Day 2: Conditioning + Mobility**
- **Day 3: Strength + Core**
- **Day 4: Conditioning + Core**
- **Day 5: Full-body Circuit (Hybrid)**
- **Day 6: Active Recovery or Rest**
- **Day 7: Complete Rest**

This split balances intensity and recovery, allowing your body to adapt while avoiding burnout. You'll rotate between strength-focused sessions, cardio conditioning, core development, and tactical-style circuits that mimic the demands of military fitness.

Choose Your Level

Each workout will include progressions for three fitness levels:

- **Level 1 – Recruit (Beginner):** If you're new to training or returning after a long break.

- **Level 2 – Operator (Intermediate):** You've been training but want to step up.

- **Level 3 – Elite (Advanced):** You're already fit and ready for high performance.

Start at the level you can complete with solid form. You can always move up when you've earned it.

Gear Needed (Optional)

While the plan is bodyweight-based, the following gear is helpful:

- Pull-up bar (or access to a sturdy bar/tree)
- Backpack with weight (10–20 kg)
- Resistance bands
- Timer or stopwatch
- Notebook (or app) for tracking

If you don't have these, no problem. You'll find bodyweight alternatives throughout the program.

Tracking & Progression

Every rep matters. Every second counts.

Track your performance daily — reps, time, rounds completed, rest times, and how you felt. Use the tracking sheet in the appendix or a simple notebook.

Each week, the volume or difficulty increases slightly. You're not just going through the motions — you're actively leveling up.

Warm-Up Protocol (Before Every Workout)

Start every session with this short warm-up to prime your body:

- Jumping Jacks – 1 minute
- Arm Circles (Forward/Backward) – 30 seconds each
- World's Greatest Stretch – 1 min per side
- Air Squats – 15 reps
- Inchworms – 5 reps
- Plank Hold – 30 seconds

Take 3–5 minutes, get your blood flowing, and mentally flip the switch: it's time to train.

WEEK 1 – BUILD THE BASE

This is where you build structure, learn the movement patterns, and create consistency. Focus on quality, not speed.

Day 1 – Strength + Core
Push-ups – 3x8 (Recruit) / 3x15 (Operator) / 4x20 (Elite)
Air Squats – 3x15 / 3x25 / 4x30
Glute Bridges – 3x10 / 3x15 / 4x20
Plank – 3x20s / 3x30s / 3x45s

Day 2 – Conditioning + Mobility
Jog/Walk Intervals – 20 min (1 min jog, 1 min walk)
Mobility: Shoulder circles, hip openers, T-spine rotations – 5 minutes

Day 3 – Strength + Core

Incline Push-ups / Regular / Diamond – 3 sets
Walking Lunges – 2x10 (each leg) / 3x12 / 4x15
Bird-Dogs – 2x10 / 3x10 / 3x12
Side Plank – 2x20s / 3x30s / 3x40s per side

Day 4 – Conditioning + Core
High Knees – 30s

Bodyweight Squats – 20 reps
Mountain Climbers – 30s
Repeat circuit x 3 (Recruit) / 4 (Operator) / 5 (Elite)
Core: Hollow Hold – 3x20s / 3x30s / 3x45s

Day 5 – Hybrid Circuit (Full Body)
3–4 rounds of:

- 10 Push-ups

- 10 Squats

- 30s Plank

- 10 Jumping Jacks
  Rest 30–60s between rounds

Day 6 – Active Recovery
Easy walk, mobility, light stretching – 20–30 minutes

Day 7 – Rest

Don't forget that resting is as important as training.

WEEK 2 – INCREASE THE LOAD

Add reps. Reduce rest. The body adapts through demand.

Workouts increase in complexity — some movements become harder, and you'll feel the difference. Stick with the plan.

WEEK 3 – CONTROL & CONSISTENCY

This week focuses on clean movement and bracing under tension. You're now deep into building the foundation — don't rush.

Plank holds get longer. Push-ups become tighter. Conditioning gets snappier.

WEEK 4 – INTENSITY SHIFT

Midpoint of the program.

Expect higher output: faster circuits, tougher progressions, more reps. Start incorporating a weighted backpack if you're ready.

Push through mental fatigue — this week is about showing yourself what you're capable of.

WEEK 5 – STRESS TEST

Every session gets harder.

You'll add short sprints to conditioning work, reduce rest times, and push the limits of your endurance.

If Week 1 was about forming a habit, Week 5 is about proving your resilience.

WEEK 6 – MISSION READY

This is the final week. The challenge is full-volume and full-effort.

You'll perform the most difficult version of every movement you've practiced — and you'll complete a final full-body assessment at the end.

Keep your journal close. Reflect daily. This is where the work pays off.

Scaling and Substitutions

If you can't do a movement (yet), swap it:

- No pull-up bar? Do rows under a table or backpack pulls.
- Too tired for high-impact cardio? Walk fast on an incline or ruck.
- Can't jump? Do step-backs or static lunges instead.

Modify intelligently — but don't skip.

When to Rest

You're training five days a week. But if your body really needs some rest: just take it. The mission isn't about breaking yourself. It's about becoming stronger.

Signs you need rest:

- Poor sleep
- Sore joints
- Mood changes
- Significant drop in performance

If needed, swap Day 6 (active recovery) with an earlier day. Just don't disappear. Adjust — and return. Remember: discipline over motivation.

Final Assessment

At the end of Week 6, repeat your starting assessment from Chapter 4.

- Push-ups in 2 minutes
- 1.5-mile run or equivalent
- Max squat reps
- Core hold (plank or hollow hold)
- Mobility check (hip, shoulder range)

Compare your results. You'll be surprised at what's changed — not just physically, but mentally.

Beyond the 6 Weeks

This plan isn't the finish line.

It's the start of your next level. After 6 weeks, you can:

- Repeat the plan at a higher level
- Shift focus (strength or fat loss plan in Chapter 6)
- Add gear, weight, or new environments

- Build a new 6-week mission

This book gives you the system. Now it's your job to lead yourself forward.

Mission Complete? Not Yet

You've survived six weeks of consistent, structured, real training. You've learned discipline, built strength, developed endurance, and sharpened your mind.

But here's the truth: the real mission never ends.

Keep showing up. Keep improving. Keep leading yourself.

You're not a recruit anymore.

You're a soldier in your own life.

7. Targeted Tracks for Fat Loss and Strength

Not every mission has the same objective. Some of you are here to drop body fat. Others want to build raw, usable strength. Some want both, but are prioritizing one path for now. This chapter gives you the tools to adapt the 6-week Tactical Fitness Plan to your specific goal. You don't need a new program — you need to apply the right adjustments to the structure you already have.

Choosing the Right Track

Before diving into split charts or workout tweaks, you need clarity: what is your mission right now?

If your goal is fat loss, your training must emphasize calorie expenditure, metabolic stress, and muscular endurance. That means circuits, short rest periods, and high movement density. You'll burn more, move more, and sweat more — all while preserving muscle mass.

If your goal is strength, your focus shifts. You need to apply progressive resistance, emphasize quality reps over quantity, and give your body the rest it needs to rebuild. The training is still hard — but it's different. It's slower, more focused, and more demanding on your nervous system.

Whichever path you choose, commit fully. Six weeks is enough time to make real progress — but only if your actions are aligned with your goal.

Track 1: Fat Loss Mission Plan

Fat loss isn't just about working hard — it's about working smart. The goal is to trigger fat metabolism, maintain muscle, and prevent burnout. This isn't about starving yourself or doing endless cardio. It's about consistency, intensity, and recovery.

Weekly Structure (Fat Loss Track)

- **Monday** – Full-body Conditioning Circuit
- **Tuesday** – Mobility + Core Stability

- **Wednesday** – Full-body Strength + HIIT Finisher
- **Thursday** – Active Recovery (walk, ruck, or mobility)
- **Friday** – Metcon (Metabolic Conditioning) + Core
- **Saturday** – Long-Duration Zone 2 Cardio (ruck, jog, bike)
- **Sunday** – Full Rest

Training Notes

- Use compound movements to target multiple muscle groups at once.
- Keep rest periods short (30–60 seconds).
- Prioritize movement quality, but push your pace.
- Maintain intensity even if reps drop over time.

Nutrition Mission for Fat Loss

- **Caloric Deficit**: Eat 300–500 calories below maintenance.
- **High Protein**: Aim for 1.6–2.2 g protein per kg of bodyweight.
- **Hydration**: 2.5–3.5 liters per day.
- **Track Progress Weekly**: Waist size, visual changes, energy levels — not just scale weight.

Fat Loss Mental Tips

- You don't need to be perfect. You need to be consistent.
- Hunger ≠ progress. Focus on performance, not deprivation.
- Sleep matters — 6 hours or less kills fat loss.
- Don't chase soreness. Chase sustainability.

Fat Loss Weekly Goals

Week Goal

Week	Goal
1	Establish baseline, tighten nutrition, complete all sessions

Week Goal

Week	Goal
2	Improve circuit times, reduce unnecessary snacking
3	Increase reps in core movements, maintain deficit without fatigue
4	Shift into fat-burning zone: maximize output, review progress
5	Hold intensity, manage stress, recover hard
6	Peak effort — most consistent week, dial in performance metrics

Fat Loss Tracking Metrics

- Circuit completion time
- Resting heart rate
- Waist/hip ratio
- Sleep quality
- Mood and energy scores (1–10 scale)

Don't expect fat to fall off overnight. It doesn't. But week by week, with discipline and structure, your body will change. You'll move lighter, faster, and longer — with clarity and focus.

Track 2: Strength Mission Plan

If your mission is strength, every rep must count. Strength doesn't come from going all-out every day — it comes from intentional, progressive training with enough recovery to grow. This track is slower-paced but heavier on execution. More control, more mastery.

Weekly Structure (Strength Track)

- **Monday** – Full-body Strength (push + pull)
- **Tuesday** – Core + Mobility
- **Wednesday** – Lower Body Strength + Carries
- **Thursday** – Active Recovery (mobility, walking, stretching)
- **Friday** – Upper Body Volume + Grip Work

- **Saturday** – Optional Conditioning or Skills (slow ruck, swimming, climbing)
- **Sunday** – Full Rest

Training Notes

- Perform exercises at a slower tempo (e.g., 3s down, 1s pause).
- Use weighted backpacks, vests, or resistance bands if available.
- Focus on form and full range of motion.
- Rest 60–120 seconds between sets.

Strength-Focused Movements

- Push-ups (standard, archer, decline)
- Pull-ups (assisted or strict)
- Bulgarian split squats
- Ruck squats and step-ups
- Weighted carries (farmer, overhead, front rack)
- Plank variations (RKC, side, loaded)

Nutrition Mission for Strength

- **Slight Surplus**: 200–300 calories above maintenance.
- **Protein First**: Same as fat loss (1.6–2.2 g/kg BW).
- **Post-Workout Nutrition**: Prioritize protein + carbs.
- **Hydration and Electrolytes**: Especially if you're adding load or sweating more.

Strength Mental Tips

- Keep a log — strength is about numbers and tracking.
- Stop chasing fatigue — chase progress.
- Focus on tension and technique.
- Don't skip rest days. Growth happens during recovery.

Strength Weekly Goals

Week Goal

1   Establish baseline: max reps, form check, movement prep

2   Increase volume on major lifts, track tempo

3   Progress to harder variations or add load

4   Deload slightly if needed — manage fatigue

5   Peak week: max volume without failure

6   Performance test: max reps, holds, and carries

Strength Tracking Metrics

- Max push-ups in 2 minutes
- Max pull-ups or hangs
- Weighted carry distance
- Time under tension (for planks, holds, etc.)
- Weekly training load and progress

Strength is about precision. Not just lifting more, but lifting better. You're not just building muscle — you're training your nervous system to command more force. That's a skill. And it takes patience.

Switching Tracks Mid-Mission

Sometimes you'll start with one goal and shift to another. That's fine — as long as it's intentional. If you began on the fat loss track and realize you're under-recovering, consider moving to strength. If you've built a strong base and now want to shred down, you can pivot to fat loss — but reset your expectations. Changing the mission resets the clock.

Before switching, ask:

- Why am I changing?
- Have I completed at least 3 full weeks?

- Am I making excuses or responding to data?

Track first. Decide second.

What If You Want Both?

It's possible to build strength and lose fat at the same time — especially if you're new to training or returning from a break. But results will come more slowly. You can blend the two tracks (strength days + conditioning finishers), but only if you recover properly. Sleep, nutrition, and stress control must be locked in. We'll cover this part in the following chapters.

For most people, it's better to choose one track, commit to it for six weeks, and then switch. You'll see better results and clearer progress.

Sample Hybrid Week (Advanced Only)

- **Monday** – Strength Focus (push + pull)
- **Tuesday** – Mobility + Core
- **Wednesday** – Conditioning Circuit (fat loss track)
- **Thursday** – Rest
- **Friday** – Lower Body Strength
- **Saturday** – Ruck or Long Cardio
- **Sunday** – Rest

Use this only if you've trained consistently for 6+ months and know your recovery capacity.

Final Briefing

Mission success is built on alignment — aligning your training, nutrition, rest, and mindset with your goal. The general 6-week tactical plan gave you the structure. This chapter gives you precision. Whether your target is fat loss or strength, execute with clarity and commitment.

8. Fuel the Mission: Tactical Nutrition for Performance

If your training is the engine, nutrition is the fuel. You can run the hardest workouts, do the toughest circuits, and stay consistent for weeks, but if you're eating the wrong way, your progress will stall. Not because you're weak. Not because you lack effort. But because your body isn't being given the resources it needs to grow, recover, or burn fat effectively.

This chapter gives you a clear, no-nonsense strategy for eating like a soldier. That means simplicity, discipline, and consistency. No counting almonds. No restrictive diets. Just solid tactical eating that supports performance.

Whether your mission is fat loss, strength, or endurance, this chapter will help you eat to win.

The Tactical Nutrition Pyramid

Not all nutrition advice is created equal. People tend to get distracted by details — supplements, timing, or meal names — while ignoring the foundations. That's why this system is built as a pyramid, with the most important elements at the base.

Here's how to prioritize:

1. **Calories** – Your total energy intake. No matter what your goal is — fat loss, strength, or endurance — total calories matter most.

2. **Macros** – Protein, carbohydrates, and fats. Once your calories are dialed in, your macronutrient ratio will shape how your body adapts to the training.

3. **Food Quality** – Once calories and macros are on point, you focus on nutrient-dense, minimally processed foods for performance, digestion, and long-term health.

4. **Timing** – When you eat matters, but it's a distant fourth. You don't need perfect timing. You need consistency.

5. **Supplements** – These come very last. They're only effective when the rest of the pyramid is already in place.

When in doubt, return to the base: get your calories and protein right, and most of your progress will follow.

Caloric Balance: The Core of Change

Calories are energy. Eat more than your body needs = weight gain. Eat less = weight loss. Eat roughly what you burn = maintenance.

That's the principle — simple, but not always easy in practice. Most people either underestimate what they eat or overestimate how much they burn. This program uses a **practical estimation** to get you in the right ballpark.

Step 1: Estimate Your Baseline Needs

Use this simple formula based on your bodyweight:

- **Fat Loss:** 24–26 kcal per kg of body weight
- **Maintenance/Endurance:** 28–30 kcal/kg
- **Muscle Gain/Strength:** 32–36 kcal/kg

Example (80 kg person):

- Fat loss: ~2,000 kcal/day
- Maintenance: ~2,400 kcal/day
- Strength: ~2,800 kcal/day

These aren't perfect — they're your **starting point**. Use them to build your plan, then adjust weekly based on progress. If you're not seeing results after 10–14 days, recalculate.

Macronutrient Breakdown

Now that you have a calorie target, you need to split it into macros. Macronutrients (macros) are the nutrients your body needs in large amounts: **protein, carbohydrates**, and **fats**.

Here's how to break it down for tactical goals:

1. Protein – Your Recovery and Repair Macro

Protein supports muscle maintenance, repair, and growth. It's also the most satiating macro — it helps control hunger.

- **Goal:** 1.6–2.2g per kg of body weight
- **Example (80 kg person):** 130–175g/day

This should be consistent whether your goal is fat loss or muscle building. You can't "train hard" if your muscles don't recover.

Best protein sources:

- Lean meat, fish, eggs
- Cottage cheese, Greek yogurt
- Tofu, tempeh, lentils
- Whey protein
-

2. Carbs – The Tactical Fuel

Carbs are not your enemy — they're your ally. Your body uses carbs as its **primary energy source** during high-intensity training. Without them, you'll feel sluggish, foggy, and drained.

- **Goal range:** 2–6g per kg of body weight
  - Lower end (2–3g/kg): Fat loss
  - Higher end (4–6g/kg): Strength/endurance goals
- **Example (80 kg person):**
  - Fat loss: 160–240g/day
  - Endurance: 320–480g/day

Best sources:

- Oats, rice, potatoes, quinoa
- Fruit, beans, legumes
- Whole wheat pasta, bread (in moderation)
- Vegetables (fiber + micronutrients)

Choose complex carbs that release energy steadily — they keep you fueled without crashing.

3. Fats – The Hormonal Anchor

Dietary fat supports hormone production, vitamin absorption, and long-term satiety. You don't want to go too low, especially if you're training hard.

- **Goal:** 0.8–1g per kg of body weight
- **Example (80 kg person):** 65–80g/day

Good fat sources:

- Eggs, fatty fish, olive oil, nuts
- Avocados, seeds, full-fat yogurt

Avoid trans fats and highly processed oils. Stick to whole, natural fat sources.

Sample Macro Distribution

Here are two sample daily setups:

Fat Loss – 2,000 kcal/day target (80 kg)

- Protein: 160g (640 kcal)
- Carbs: 180g (720 kcal)
- Fat: 72g (640 kcal)

Strength – 2,800 kcal/day target (80 kg)

- Protein: 170g (680 kcal)
- Carbs: 360g (1,440 kcal)
- Fat: 75g (680 kcal)

Nutrient Quality: Fuel, Not Just Calories

All calories are not created equal. 500 kcal of fried junk and 500 kcal of lean chicken with sweet potato will have very different effects on your energy, digestion, recovery, and hunger.

That said, you don't need to eat like a monk. The **80/20 Rule** is your guide: eat 80% whole, nutrient-dense foods, and give yourself 20% flexibility.

✅ Choose:

- Lean meats, eggs, legumes, tofu
- Fresh vegetables and fruits
- Whole grains and tubers
- Nuts, seeds, healthy oils

❌ Limit:

- Deep-fried foods
- Soda, ultra-processed snacks
- Sugary breakfast cereals
- Alcohol (slows recovery and drains energy)

This isn't about perfection. It's about intention. Make food choices that support your mission. Be strict with yourself, but remember that your diet needs to be sustainable.

Meal Timing and Structure

When you eat matters — but not as much as what and how much you eat.

Still, having a structured eating schedule helps maintain energy levels, support recovery, and avoid overeating.

3–5 Meal Framework

Depending on your daily routine, aim for:

- 3 larger meals
- OR
- 3 meals + 1–2 snacks

Spread protein evenly throughout the day to improve recovery and muscle retention. Try to avoid skipping meals or eating everything late at night.

Pre-Workout Fuel

Eat 1–2 hours before training. Focus on carbs and protein.

- Example:
    - Oats + banana + Greek yogurt
    - Rice + chicken breast + veggies
    - Apple + protein shake

Avoid large, fat-heavy meals right before training — they slow digestion. If you want to lose weight, 0% fat Greek yogurt is a solid option for healthy proteins with very low calories.

Post-Workout Recovery

Eat within 1–2 hours after training. Focus on fast-digesting carbs and lean protein.

- Example:
    - Rice + lean meat + veggies
    - Whole wheat wrap + eggs
    - Protein shake + banana

The post-workout window doesn't need to be exact, but it should be consistent. You just stressed your system — now fuel the repair process.

Eating Clean Without Overthinking

Nutrition can easily become overwhelming: calorie counting, meal prep, macros, tracking apps, cheat meals — the list goes on. But tactical nutrition isn't about creating stress. It's about building a system that works under pressure — just like everything else in your training.

If you followed the framework from Part 1, you already understand what to eat and how much. Now it's time to make it sustainable. That means choosing structure over chaos, repetition over novelty, and systems over hype.

The goal is simple: Remove friction. Eat for performance. Keep it simple.

A good tactical meal:

- Has a protein source
- Includes a slow-digesting carb or fiber
- Uses some healthy fat
- Is fast to prepare or batch-cook
- Can be repeated or modified easily

Example Meals:
- **Breakfast:** 4 eggs, oats with fruit, black coffee
- **Lunch:** Grilled chicken, quinoa, steamed spinach, olive oil
- **Dinner:** Ground turkey, lentils, roasted vegetables
- **Snack:** Greek yogurt + banana + 10 almonds
- **Field Option:** Tuna pouch + instant rice + carrots
-

Meal Prep = Strategic Discipline

The easiest way to stick to a performance diet is to cook ahead whenever you have some free time. Prep two or three meals in bulk — protein, carbs, and veg — then portion them into containers. You can rotate seasonings and sauces to avoid boredom. Spices are a great way to make food more exciting without exceeding your targeted calories.

Batch-cooking not only saves time, but it also makes your choices automatic. You're not scrambling to "figure out" dinner after a long day or a tough session — it's ready. In tactical training, this is the difference between fueling the mission and falling behind. Prep once, eat four times.

Budget-Friendly Tactical Eating

You don't need $15 organic smoothies or custom meal kits to eat well. Some of the best performance foods are affordable, shelf-stable, and simple.

Here's how to build a high-performance diet on a budget:
- Buy in bulk: oats, rice, lentils, beans, frozen veggies

- Choose whole eggs over pricey protein bars
- Get frozen over fresh when prices spike
- Shop store-brand Greek yogurt, cottage cheese, tuna
- Cook with base ingredients, not packaged meals

Clean eating doesn't need to be expensive. It needs to be consistent and well-organized.

Hydration: The Forgotten Performance Tool

Most people walk around underhydrated, then wonder why they feel tired, slow, or foggy. Your muscles are 70% water. Your brain? About 75%. Even a 2% drop in hydration can impair focus and endurance.

Hydration strategy:

- Start your day with 500ml of water
- Drink 2.5–4L per day, more in heat or high-output training
- Add salt or electrolytes if sweating heavily (sodium, potassium, magnesium)
- Limit energy drinks — rely on water, black coffee, or tea

Pro tip: Cold water, fast sips before and after training improve performance and recovery.

Tactical Eating Under Stress or in the Field

Some days you won't be home. Maybe you're working long shifts, on the move, or in unpredictable situations. That's where tactical nutrition earns its name: **adaptability over perfection**.

Packable, shelf-stable tactical fuel:

- Tuna or salmon pouches
- Instant oats
- Rice cakes
- Dried fruit + nuts
- Peanut butter
- Protein powder

- Jerky
- Hard-boiled eggs
- Protein bars (look for 15g+ protein, low sugar)

Keep these in your ruck, backpack, or glove box. You don't skip training because conditions aren't ideal — treat your nutrition the same way.

Eating for Fat Loss: Strategic Discipline

Fat loss doesn't mean starvation. It means staying slightly below maintenance calories (typically 300–500 kcal/day), keeping protein high, and staying consistent for 6+ weeks.

- Use lower-calorie carbs (vegetables, legumes, fruit) to stay full
- Drink lots of water and eat slowly
- Stick to simple meals repeated often
- Avoid liquid calories (soda, alcohol, cream)
- Prepare for hunger: it's part of the process

Example Day (Fat Loss – 2,000 kcal target):

- Breakfast: 3 eggs + veggies + oats (400 kcal)
- Lunch: Lentils + brown rice + spinach (500 kcal)
- Snack: Greek yogurt + berries (200 kcal)
- Dinner: Chicken breast + sweet potato + broccoli (600 kcal)
- Post-workout shake: Whey protein + banana (300 kcal)

Track your intake (apps like MyFitnessPal work well), but don't obsess. What matters most is consistency week to week.

Eating for Strength or Muscle Gain

To build muscle or strength, you need to be in a slight calorie surplus (200–400 kcal/day) and prioritize progressive training and quality sleep. Protein must stay high, but carbs go higher to support training volume.

- Eat 4–5 meals daily, evenly spaced

- Prioritize post-workout recovery (protein + carbs)
- Include more dense carbs (rice, pasta, bread, oats)
- Avoid "dirty bulking" — stay lean and intentional

Example Day (Muscle Gain – 2,800 kcal):

- Breakfast: 4 eggs + oats + peanut butter + banana (700 kcal)
- Snack: Cottage cheese + apple + almonds (400 kcal)
- Lunch: Chicken breast + rice + olive oil + veggies (700 kcal)
- Snack: Protein shake + rice cakes (300 kcal)
- Dinner: Ground beef + pasta + spinach (700 kcal)

Monitor bodyweight weekly — aim for 0.25–0.5 kg gained per week.

The Tactical Meal Kit: Reusable Strategy

To simplify everything, here's the formula to build any tactical meal:

1. **Choose a Protein:**
   o Chicken, turkey, eggs, tofu, fish, whey, cottage cheese
2. **Add a Carb Source:**
   o Rice, oats, pasta, quinoa, beans, lentils, sweet potato
3. **Add Veggies or Fiber:**
   o Spinach, carrots, broccoli, bell peppers, kale, onions
4. **Add Fat (Optional):**
   o Olive oil, avocado, seeds, nuts
5. **Season and Repeat**
   o Use spices, garlic, herbs, lemon, vinegar, mustard

You can build 30+ different meals using the same 10 ingredients — no need for new recipes every day.

Supplements: Minimal, Purposeful

Supplements are not shortcuts — but a few are worth considering after your diet is solid.

Useful Options:

- **Whey protein** – Convenient, fast-digesting
- **Creatine monohydrate** – Strength, power, and recovery
- **Vitamin D** – If you're not in the sun
- **Electrolytes** – Especially in heat or endurance training
- **Caffeine (in moderation)** – For performance, focus

Skip the fat burners, detox teas, and overpriced blends. Train hard, eat clean, sleep deep — that's your real stack.

Realistic but Relentless

You're not a robot. There will be days when meals get skipped, your schedule gets wrecked, or your motivation dips. That's not failure — that's nothing but real life. The mission is adaptation, not perfection. Missed a meal? Hit the next one. Ate poorly on the weekend? Get back on plan Monday. Didn't prep? Make the cleanest choice available.

Just like your workouts, your nutrition is a discipline. You don't rise to the occasion. You fall to the level of your systems.

9. Tactical Recovery

Your progress doesn't happen while you're training — it happens while you recover. That's not a motivational slogan. It's a physiological fact.

In military training, soldiers are pushed hard, often beyond what the average person would tolerate. But the best programs also know when to pull back. Recovery is not weakness. It's part of the plan. And if you neglect it, your results will stall, your risk of injury will rise, and your energy will crash.

This chapter is a field manual for understanding, managing, and optimizing recovery — physically, neurologically, and hormonally. If training is your offense, recovery is your defense. You need both to win.

The Physiology of Recovery

Training creates a stress response in your body — a controlled breakdown of tissue, energy systems, and central nervous system (CNS) output. This breakdown is a *stimulus*. If followed by recovery, the body adapts and grows stronger. If not, you accumulate fatigue, stress hormones (like cortisol), and eventually overtrain or burn out.

Recovery is when:

- Muscle fibers rebuild stronger.

- Energy stores (like glycogen) are replenished.

- Hormones like testosterone and growth hormone rebalance.

- Inflammation is resolved.

- The nervous system restores balance between sympathetic ("fight or flight") and parasympathetic ("rest and digest").

Ignoring this process doesn't make you hardcore — it makes you reckless.

Key Components of Recovery

There are four main pillars of recovery:

1. **Sleep**

2. **Nutrition**

3. **Movement & Circulation**

4. **Nervous System Regulation**

We've already addressed nutrition in depth, so this chapter focuses on the other three.

1. Sleep: The Foundation of Recovery

No supplement, no foam roller, and no "hack" replaces what sleep does. It's the most anabolic (rebuilding) and anti-catabolic (anti-breakdown) time your body has. Without 7–9 hours of quality sleep, your training suffers — regardless of your discipline.

What Happens During Sleep:

- Growth hormone surges during deep sleep (especially in the first few hours).

- Muscle tissue is rebuilt.

- The brain consolidates motor learning and memory — crucial for movement pattern retention.

- Cortisol (stress hormone) is reduced.

- The immune system resets.

Tactical Sleep Targets:

- **Goal**: 7.5 to 9 hours per night

- **Minimum**: 6 hours (short term), but not sustainable

- **Nap protocol**: If sleep is missed, a 20–30 min power nap can help restore alertness and reduce stress

Sleep Optimization Strategies:

- Go to bed and wake up at the same time — even on weekends.

- Block blue light from screens 1 hour before bed (use apps like f.lux or blue-blocking glasses).

- Keep your room dark and cool (16–19°C / 60–67°F).

- Avoid caffeine within 8 hours of sleep.

- Don't train hard right before bed — allow 2+ hours for adrenaline to come down.

Sleep isn't just a quantity game. Quality matters. If you're in bed for 8 hours but wake up 5 times, you're not recovering properly. Track your sleep with apps or wearables if needed — not obsessively, but for awareness.

2. Movement & Circulation: Active Recovery

Some trainees mistakenly associate "rest" with complete inactivity. But the goal of recovery is *circulation*, not stillness. Low-intensity movement helps:

- Flush metabolic waste products

- Deliver oxygen and nutrients to tissue

- Reduce muscle soreness (DOMS)

- Improve joint mobility

- Reset movement patterns disrupted by hard training

This is where **active recovery** comes in.

Active Recovery Methods:

- **Walks** (30–45 minutes, low pace)

- **Mobility circuits** (light bodyweight flows, yoga-based drills)

- **Biking or swimming** (low intensity, steady pace)

- **Foam rolling or trigger point work** (if tightness is present)

- **Joint mobility drills** (shoulders, hips, spine, ankles)

Use your rest days wisely. A 30-minute walk or mobility session will often speed up recovery more than lying on the couch. Blood flow heals tissue. Inactivity slows it down.

If a specific area feels tight or sore, prioritize low-intensity movement through that area rather than stretching it cold. Never force mobility on inflammation — the goal is to nourish, not stress.

3. Nervous System Regulation: Downshifting

One of the most overlooked recovery tools isn't physical — it's neurological.

Every training session activates your **sympathetic nervous system**: the high-alert, adrenaline-fueled, "fight or flight" response. This is necessary to push hard. But if you stay there too long — if you never return to **parasympathetic** mode — your body never truly recovers.

Signs your nervous system is out of balance:

- Restless sleep
- Elevated resting heart rate
- Mood swings or irritability
- Poor appetite or digestion
- Reduced performance despite consistent training

Tools to Downshift the Nervous System:

- **Box breathing**: Inhale 4 seconds → hold 4 → exhale 4 → hold 4. Repeat for 5+ minutes.

- **Cold exposure**: Short, controlled exposure (30–90 seconds) post-workout or in the morning — resets stress tolerance.

- **Mindful walking**: No phone, no podcast. Just awareness of breath and environment.

- **Journaling**: Dumping mental stress on paper reduces internal pressure.

- **Stretching with breath**: Combine mobility work with long, nasal exhalations.

If you can shift your body *out* of high-stress mode post-workout, you'll recover faster, sleep deeper, and train harder the next day.

Tactical Rest Days: How to Use Them

You don't "earn" rest days by collapsing from exhaustion. You plan them into the system — because they're part of the system.

This program includes **1–2 rest or active recovery days per week**. Here's how to use them effectively.

Active Recovery Day Example:

- 15–20 minutes of full-body mobility (spine, hips, shoulders)
- 30-minute walk or light bike ride
- 5–10 minutes of core activation (planks, dead bugs, bird-dogs)
- Hydration + high-protein meals + low stimulation (no phone scrolling binges)

Full Rest Day (Complete Reset):

- Sleep in (if possible)
- Hydrate aggressively
- Focus on protein and micronutrient-rich foods
- Stretch or foam roll only if needed
- No training, no strain, no guilt

Both are valid. Choose based on your body's feedback. If you feel beat down — take the full rest. If you just feel stiff — do the active recovery.

Recovery Is Training: Log It Like You Log Workouts

One of the best ways to make recovery intentional is to **track it**, just like your workouts.

Here's what you can log daily or weekly:

Metric	Why It Matters
Sleep hours	Indicates recovery capacity
Resting heart rate	Elevated = possible stress or illness
Soreness levels	Chronic = under-recovery
Mood/energy rating	Low = potential overtraining or underfueling
Training performance	Declining = red flag

You don't need to obsess over numbers — but if you're stalling in progress, this data often holds the answer.

Pro tip: If your resting heart rate is up by more than 7–10 bpm for two consecutive mornings, consider a rest day.

Avoiding Overtraining

True overtraining is rare — but *under-recovering* is common. Here are the signs to watch for:

- Decreased performance despite training harder
- Constant fatigue, even after a rest day
- Sleep disruptions
- Mood changes or irritability
- Frequent illnesses or injuries
- Loss of motivation or burnout

If you experience 3 or more of these for over a week, reduce intensity and prioritize sleep, food, and light movement. The goal isn't to be fragile — it's to stay functional.

Supplemental Recovery Tools: Do They Work?

Not essential — but worth considering if your basics are dialed in.

Tool	Benefit	Worth It?
Magnesium (citrate/glycinate)	Aids sleep, muscle relaxation	☑ Yes
Creatine Monohydrate	Supports strength, cognitive function	☑ Yes
Omega-3 (EPA/DHA)	Reduces inflammation, joint health	☑ Yes
Foam Rolling	Temporary relief improves mobility	☑ Yes (short term)
Massage gun	Can aid circulation	Optional
Ice baths	Nervous system reset, cold shock benefit	☑ Yes (short)
Saunas	Promotes circulation, detox, and CNS balance	☑ Yes

Supplements should **support** recovery, not replace bad habits. Start with sleep, food, and hydration. The rest is a bonus.

Final Notes on Recovery

Recovery isn't soft. It's smart. Soldiers don't train to collapse. They train to repeat, to endure, and to remain operational under pressure — day after day.

The goal isn't to do one great workout and burn out. It's to build a body and mind that can handle consistent, sustained performance.

So treat your recovery like a mission: Plan it. Track it. Adjust it. Respect it. The work doesn't end when the training stops. That's where the rebuilding begins.

10. Field Conditions & Minimalist Tactics

You might now always find a gym. You might not always find perfect weather. But it will work out if you have the right plan.

This chapter focuses on one of the most important tactical fitness skills: the ability to **train anywhere**, anytime, under any condition. Whether you're deployed, traveling, stuck in a hotel room, or working with limited space and gear, the mission doesn't stop. The most effective soldiers and athletes aren't the ones who wait for the right conditions — they adapt, improvise, and keep moving forward.

Let's break down how to build workouts, progress, and stay accountable with **minimal equipment and maximum efficiency**.

Environments You Can Train In

It's easy to fall into the trap of thinking that training must be tied to a specific place — the gym, the track, the park. But real tactical fitness means being ready anywhere. Here's how to train in different environments:

1. Indoors (Hotel, Apartment, Barracks Room)

- Space required: 2x2 meters
- Use bodyweight movements like push-ups, squats, lunges, planks, and burpees
- Use furniture (chair, bed, backpack) as props for dips, elevated push-ups, or rows
- Do circuits or EMOM (Every Minute on the Minute) workouts to maximize time and effort
- Keep noise low with tempo control if needed (slow, controlled reps)

2. Outdoors (Park, Field, Trail, Beach)

- Use benches, stairs, trees, or playground bars
- Sand and uneven surfaces build balance and coordination

- Carry rocks, logs, or sandbags for resistance

- Add sprints, shuttles, crawling drills, or hill runs

3. Travel / Deployment

- Pack a jump rope, resistance bands, or TRX-style straps (lightweight, versatile)

- Use a rucksack filled with clothing, books, or water bottles

- Stick to bodyweight and mobility sessions when gear is limited

- Save workouts on your phone or notebook — don't rely on Wi-Fi

4. Emergency / No-Time Situations

- Have a 10-minute go-to session: Example:
    o 10 push-ups
    o 15 squats
    o 10 lunges
    o 20 mountain climbers
    o Repeat x 3

- Do something — even 5 minutes of high-effort training maintains the habit

The Minimal Gear Kit

You don't need much to train effectively. Here's a list of compact, inexpensive gear that expands your options:

- **Backpack/Ruck** – Load it with books or bottles and use it for loaded carries, squats, lunges, or rucking

- **Resistance Bands** – Perfect for rows, curls, press, shoulder rehab, and mobility work

- **Pull-up Bar (doorway or portable)** – Game-changer for upper-body training
- **Jump Rope** – Excellent conditioning tool, great for coordination and footwork
- **Yoga Mat or Towel** – Protects knees/back, helps with ground-based work

Optional extras:

- Suspension trainer (TRX or similar)
- Ab wheel
- Sandbag or duffel bag (for DIY strength)

How to Structure Minimalist Workouts

Even without a gym, you still need a balanced training structure. The three pillars of tactical fitness still apply: strength, conditioning, and mobility. Here's how to build effective sessions in any location:

1. Strength Focused (Bodyweight or Light Load)
Choose 3–4 movements. Do 3–5 rounds, focusing on control and full range of motion.

Example – Strength Session (30 min):

- Push-ups x 12
- Bulgarian Split Squats x 10/leg (use chair or couch)
- Backpack Rows x 12
- Plank to Push-up x 10
- Rest 60–90 sec between rounds

Modify reps to fit your level.

2. Conditioning Focused (High Intensity)
Keep it simple, fast, and hard. Use time-based or rep-based circuits.

Example – Conditioning Circuit (20 min):

- Jump Squats x 15
- Push-ups x 15
- Mountain Climbers x 30
- Burpees x 10
- Repeat for 4–5 rounds with minimal rest

Or:

EMOM (Every Minute on the Minute) for 10–15 min

- Minute 1: 15 push-ups
- Minute 2: 20 squats
- Minute 3: 15 sit-ups
- Repeat

3. Core + Mobility (Low Impact / Active Recovery)

Example – Core & Mobility Session:

- Dead Bug x 10
- Side Plank (30s/side)
- Bird Dog x 10
- World's Greatest Stretch x 5/side
- Downward Dog to Cobra x 5
- Repeat 2–3 rounds

Use this on rest days, while traveling, or when you're low on energy.

Training Without a Timer or Tracker

If you don't have your phone, app, or watch — that's not an excuse. Use **rounds** or **breathing** to gauge effort.

- Count sets and reps with matchsticks, coins, or rocks

- Use the sun/shadow position or the number of songs on your playlist
- Train until your breathing hits 6–7 out of 10 (moderate effort) or 9 out of 10 (hard)
- Repeat workouts weekly to track improvement without tech

How to Progress Without Equipment

You can still progress without weights. Here's how:

1. Reps & Sets – Increase reps, add rounds, reduce rest
2. Tempo – Slow down (e.g., 3-second descent, 1-second pause, fast up)
3. Angles – Make push-ups harder by elevating feet or switching to a diamond grip
4. Range of Motion – Use deeper squats or deficit push-ups
5. Density – Complete the same work in less time (or more work in the same time)

No-Excuse Scenarios and How to Handle Them

Situation	Solution
Tiny space	Do vertical exercises (squats, push-ups, planks)
No time	5–10 min high-effort circuit
Low energy	Mobility + light core work
Injury	Train around it: upper vs lower body, isometrics, rehab drills
No gear	Bodyweight + backpack + gravity
Rain or cold	Indoor drills or layer up and go
Traveling	Use a saved list of go-to sessions
Boredom	Change environment, music, or format

When You Miss a Day: Recovery or Restart

You're human. Travel, emergencies, and long hours happen. If you miss a session:

- Don't overcompensate with double sessions
- Do a short high-effort workout to "reset"
- Resume your plan where you left off
- Log what happened, so you can improve next time

Fitness is a long game. What matters is persistence.

Train Like You Might Be Deployed Tomorrow

Soldiers can't depend on gym memberships or ideal training environments. Neither should you. That's why field-ready fitness is a mindset as much as it is a method.

Train to be able to function — not just perform.

Whether you're in a crowded apartment or halfway up a mountain, your body is the gear. And discipline is the program.

11. Tactical Movement Library

Your workout is only as effective as your execution. That's why this chapter exists — to give you a clear, no-fluff guide to the most important movements in this tactical training system. These exercises are used throughout the program because they build real-world strength, mobility, endurance, and control.

You don't need to master all of them at once. But you do need to understand how they work, why they matter, and how to perform them correctly. Every movement here was chosen because it's scalable, functional, and relevant — whether you're training for fat loss, strength, or field readiness.

For each exercise, we'll include:

- **Purpose** – What it trains and why it matters

- **Execution** – Step-by-step form instructions

- **Common Mistakes** – What to watch out for

- **Progressions/Regressions** – How to scale up or down

Push Movements

Push movements build strength in the chest, shoulders, triceps, and core. They are essential for tasks like climbing, bracing, pushing loads, or simply getting up from the ground under control.

1. Push-Up (Standard)

Purpose:
Builds upper body and core strength with emphasis on real-world pushing capacity.

Execution:

1. Place hands slightly wider than shoulder-width apart.

2. Keep your body in a straight line from head to heels.

3. Lower your chest to the floor with control. Elbows should be at about a 45° angle from your body.

4. Press back up to the start position, fully extending the arms.

Common Mistakes:

- Letting the hips sag or pike
- Flaring elbows out too far
- Only doing half reps (not going all the way down)

Progressions:

- Elevate feet on a bench (decline push-up)
- Slow tempo (3 seconds down, 1 up)
- Add a weighted vest or backpack

Regressions:

- Hands elevated on a box or bench
- Knees on the ground
- Partial range of motion (but aim to build up)

2. Diamond Push-Up

Purpose:
Targets triceps and inner chest. Great for developing arm pushing strength under load.

Execution:

1. Form a diamond shape under your chest with your thumbs and index fingers.
2. Keep elbows tight to your sides as you lower.
3. Go down until your chest touches your hands, then press back up.

Common Mistakes:

- Hands too far forward (puts strain on shoulders)
- Dropping the hips
- Not maintaining control

Progressions:

- Slow tempo reps
- Feet elevated
- Add pause at the bottom

Regressions:

- Perform with hands slightly wider than diamond
- Incline surface (hands on a box)

3. Shoulder Tap Push-Up

Purpose:
Trains core stability and unilateral control while building pushing strength.

Execution:

1. Perform a push-up, then tap your left shoulder with your right hand.
2. Repeat with the opposite side.
3. Keep hips level throughout.

Common Mistakes:

- Rotating hips or shoulders
- Rushing the taps
- Not locking out the push-up fully

Progressions:

- Add a second tap after each rep
- Slow the tempo for both push-up and tap
- Add a push-up clap before tapping (advanced)

Regressions:

- Do shoulder taps in a plank instead of after push-ups
- Reduce total reps and focus on control

4. Pike Push-Up

Purpose:
Focuses on shoulder and upper chest strength. Useful for building toward handstand push-ups.

Execution:

1. Start in a downward dog position — hips high, feet flat.

2. Bend your elbows and lower your head toward the floor between your hands.

3. Push back to the start position with control.

Common Mistakes:

- Not bending elbows (turning it into a weird head-bob)

- Letting weight shift back into legs

- Rushing reps

Progressions:

- Feet on a box (elevated pike push-up)

- Handstand push-up (wall-supported)

Regressions:

- Shorten the range of motion

- Reduce volume and increase rest

Pull Movements

Pull movements train the muscles of the back, biceps, forearms, and grip — essential for climbing, dragging, lifting, and stabilizing loads. In tactical environments, pulling strength is critical for tasks like scaling walls, hauling equipment, and maintaining posture under a heavy ruck.

1. Pull-Up (Overhand Grip)

Purpose:
Develops back, shoulder, and grip strength. Foundational for upper body pulling performance.

Execution:

1. Grab a pull-up bar with palms facing away, hands slightly wider than shoulder-width.
2. Start from a dead hang — arms fully extended, feet off the ground.
3. Pull yourself up until your chin clears the bar.
4. Lower under control to a full hang. That's one rep.

Common Mistakes:

- Not reaching full extension at the bottom
- Kipping or swinging excessively
- Chin barely clearing bar without engaging full back

Progressions:

- Weighted pull-ups
- Pause at top and bottom
- Increase total sets or reduce rest

Regressions:

- Use resistance bands for assistance
- Partner-assisted pull-ups
- Perform negatives only (jump to the top, slowly lower for 3–5 sec)

2. Chin-Up (Underhand Grip)

Purpose:
Targets the biceps more heavily while still training the back and lats.

Execution:

1. Grab the bar with palms facing toward you, hands shoulder-width apart.

2. Pull yourself up until your chin clears the bar.

3. Lower slowly to a full hang.

Common Mistakes:

- Using momentum or "cheating" the bottom

- Shrugging shoulders at the top

- Reps too fast and uncontrolled

Progressions:

- Add weight with vest or backpack

- Perform slow eccentric (lowering) phase

- Pause at the top

Regressions:

- Band-assisted

- Eccentric-only reps

- Inverted rows with supinated grip

3. Bodyweight Row (Under Table or Suspension Trainer)

Purpose:
Builds horizontal pulling strength, especially for those who can't yet perform pull-ups.

Execution:

1. Lie under a sturdy table, bar, or suspension trainer with arms extended.

2. Grab the surface/handles with an overhand grip.

3. Keep your body in a straight line, heels on the floor.

4. Pull your chest to the bar or edge, then lower under control.

Common Mistakes:

- Letting hips sag
- Pulling only with arms (not engaging upper back)
- Flaring elbows too wide

Progressions:

- Elevate feet
- Slow reps (tempo 3-0-3)
- Weighted vest or backpack on chest

Regressions:

- Bend knees (easier leverage)
- Increase angle (more vertical = easier)
- Reduce reps and focus on perfect form

4. Tactical Towel Rows

Purpose:
Mimics rope climbing and enhances grip strength — crucial in field scenarios.

Execution:

1. Drape two strong towels over a pull-up bar.
2. Grab one in each hand.
3. Perform pull-ups using the towels as your grip.

Common Mistakes:

- Weak towel or bar setup — test it first
- Pulling too fast without engaging the back
- Using only arms instead of pulling from scapula

Progressions:

- Hold for time at the top
- Slow eccentrics

- Increase total reps

Regressions:
- Perform towel rows at an incline (under a low bar)
- Use one towel and one regular grip
- Train grip separately and return to this later

5. Australian Rows (Under Bar Rows)

Purpose:
Improves horizontal pulling strength, scapular control, and posture.

Execution:
1. Set a bar at waist height (or use suspension straps).
2. Lie under it with heels on the ground, arms extended.
3. Pull chest to the bar, keeping body straight.
4. Lower back to full extension.

Common Mistakes:
- Sagging hips
- Incomplete range of motion
- Rushing through reps

Progressions:
- Elevate feet
- Pause at the top
- Weighted vest

Regressions:
- Bend knees for support
- Decrease difficulty by raising bar or angle

Leg Movements

Your legs are your engine. Every mission — real or simulated — requires strong, stable, and enduring legs. Whether you're climbing stairs, sprinting to cover, or carrying a heavy load over rough terrain, your lower body needs to deliver power, control, and fatigue resistance. This section covers the foundational movements that develop leg strength and tactical readiness.

1. Bodyweight Squat

Purpose:
The cornerstone of lower-body training. Builds quad, glute, and core strength while reinforcing movement patterns.

Execution:

1. Stand with feet shoulder-width apart, toes slightly out.

2. Brace your core.

3. Lower your hips down and back like you're sitting into a chair.

4. Go as low as mobility allows (aim for thighs parallel to the ground).

5. Drive through your heels to return to standing.

Common Mistakes:

- Heels lifting off the floor
- Knees collapsing inward
- Rounding the back or leaning too far forward

Progressions:

- Jump squats
- Add a backpack or sandbag
- Pause at the bottom for 2–3 seconds

Regressions:

- Box squats (sit to a surface)
- Reduce range of motion

- Use assistance (hold onto a doorframe or TRX)

2. Split Squat

Purpose:
Improves single-leg strength, balance, and control — great for injury prevention and real-world symmetry.

Execution:

1. Stand with one foot forward, the other a few feet behind you.
2. Keep torso upright.
3. Lower your back knee toward the ground without slamming it.
4. Drive through the front heel to return to start.
5. Repeat all reps before switching legs.

Common Mistakes:

- Front knee going too far past toes
- Losing balance or tilting torso
- Not controlling the descent

Progressions:

- Bulgarian split squat (rear foot elevated)
- Weighted (vest, dumbbells, ruck)
- Jumping between reps (plyometric)

Regressions:

- Shorter range of motion
- Assisted with hands on wall or pole
- Stationary lunges

3. Step-Up (Onto Box or Bench)

Purpose:
Mimics climbing and load-bearing steps. Enhances knee and hip stability.

Execution:

1. Place one foot on a stable box or bench (knee should be around 90°).

2. Drive through the front heel to lift yourself up.

3. Avoid pushing off the back foot.

4. Lower with control. Alternate legs or complete reps on one side first.

Common Mistakes:

- Using momentum instead of control
- Box too high or unstable
- Leaning forward excessively

Progressions:

- Add weight (vest or ruck)
- Add knee drive at the top
- Step-up + reverse lunge combo

Regressions:

- Lower the height
- Use a stable platform like stairs
- Assist with hand support for balance

4. Lunge (Forward and Reverse)

Purpose:
Builds leg strength, hip mobility, and core control. Great for dynamic environments.

Execution (Forward Lunge):

1. Step forward with one leg.

2. Lower until both knees form 90° angles.

3. Push back to starting position.

4. Alternate legs.

Execution (Reverse Lunge):

1. Step backward instead of forward.

2. Lower into lunge position.

3. Push through the front foot to return.

Common Mistakes:

- Front knee collapsing inward

- Upper body leaning or twisting

- Inconsistent step size

Progressions:

- Walking lunges

- Jumping lunges

- Weighted versions

Regressions:

- Stationary lunges

- Shorter step distance

- Wall support for balance

5. Wall Sit

Purpose:
Isometric drill for building leg endurance and mental toughness.

Execution:

1. Stand with your back flat against a wall.

2. Slide down until your knees are at 90°.

3. Hold the position, keeping heels on the floor and hands off your thighs.

4. Breathe steadily. Aim for 30–60 seconds or more.

Common Mistakes:

- Knees past toes

- Sitting too low or too high
- Using arms to support weight

Progressions:

- Hold weight (backpack, plate)
- Add pulses or heel raises
- Extend one leg at a time

Regressions:

- Shorten the duration
- Partial squat hold (higher angle)
- Use a stability ball between the back and the wall

Core Movements

Your core is more than just "abs." It's the central link between your upper and lower body, and it plays a critical role in every tactical movement — sprinting, lifting, crawling, carrying, or climbing. A strong core doesn't just help you look better; it helps you move better, avoid injury, and generate power efficiently.

This section focuses on functional core exercises — movements that develop real-world strength and stability.

1. Plank (Standard and Variations)

Purpose:
Builds deep core stability, posture, and endurance. Trains your body to resist extension (arching), which protects your spine under load.

Execution (Standard Forearm Plank):

1. Elbows under shoulders, forearms parallel.
2. Legs extended, feet hip-width.
3. Keep body in a straight line — no sagging or arching.
4. Brace your core, squeeze your glutes, press heels back.
5. Hold without holding your breath.

Common Mistakes:

- Hips too high or too low
- Tension in neck or shoulders
- Not breathing properly

Progressions:

- Plank with shoulder taps
- Plank to push-up
- Ruck plank (weight on back)

Regressions:

- Knee plank
- Elevated plank (hands on bench)
- Shorter hold time with perfect form

2. Side Plank

Purpose:
Targets obliques and lateral stabilizers — essential for rotational control, spine health, and balance.

Execution:

1. Lie on one side with legs stacked.
2. Elbow directly under the shoulder.
3. Lift hips until body forms a straight line.
4. Hold or add movement (reach, raise leg, etc.)

Common Mistakes:

- Hips sagging
- Shoulders rolled forward
- Losing alignment

Progressions:

- Add leg lifts

- Weighted side plank
- Side plank with rotation

Regressions:

- Bottom knee bent and on the ground
- Shorter hold duration

3. Dead Bug

Purpose:
Trains core bracing with arm and leg movement — builds coordination and control while protecting the spine.

Execution:

1. Lie on your back, arms extended toward the ceiling, knees bent at 90°.

2. Press lower back into the ground.

3. Extend opposite arm and leg simultaneously, keeping core engaged.

4. Return and repeat on the other side.

Common Mistakes:

- Lower back lifting off the ground
- Rushing through reps
- Using momentum

Progressions:

- Add ankle weights or hold dumbbells
- Slow down reps
- Extend both legs at once

Regressions:

- Shorter leg range
- Only move arms or legs
- Keep head on the floor for support

4. Loaded Carry (Farmer's Carry / Ruck Carry)

Purpose:
Real-world core strength. Teaches posture under load, grip endurance, and breathing control.

Execution (Farmer's Carry):

1. Hold a heavy object in each hand (dumbbells, kettlebells, water jugs).
2. Stand tall, shoulders back, core tight.
3. Walk forward slowly and controlled.
4. Avoid leaning, swaying, or collapsing.

Execution (Ruck Carry):

1. Load a backpack or ruck with weight.
2. Strap it snugly on your back.
3. Walk upright — chest proud, arms relaxed.

Common Mistakes:

- Slouching forward
- Uneven gait or shuffling
- Letting weights hit your legs

Progressions:

- Heavier weights
- Longer distances
- One-sided (suitcase carry)

Regressions:

- Lighter load
- Shorter distance
- Use stairwells for added effort at low impact

5. Hollow Body Hold

Purpose:
Reinforces full-body core tension — used by gymnasts and elite tactical athletes for midline control.

Execution:

1. Lie on your back.
2. Lift shoulders and legs off the floor.
3. Arms extended overhead, lower back pressed down.
4. Hold with full tension, keeping a banana shape.

Common Mistakes:

- Arching lower back
- Letting legs drop too low
- Holding breath

Progressions:

- Add flutter kicks
- Rock slightly for dynamic challenge
- Increase duration

Regressions:

- Tuck knees in
- Keep arms at sides
- Shorter hold time

6. Bear Crawl

Purpose:
Dynamic core movement that also trains shoulder stability, hip mobility, and coordination.

Execution:

1. Start on hands and toes (knees off the floor).
2. Keep back flat, core engaged.

3. Move the opposite hand and foot forward at the same time.

4. Stay low and controlled.

Common Mistakes:

- Hips bouncing up and down

- Hands moving too far

- Losing core tension

Progressions:

- Crawl backward or sideways

- Add a resistance band around the hips

- Crawl longer distances

Regressions:

- Short distances only

- Crawl in place

- Knees down version (quadruped)

Upper Body Movements

Tactical readiness depends heavily on upper body strength — not just for lifting or pushing, but for climbing, crawling, vaulting, and pulling your body over obstacles. These movements are foundational in military fitness because they build the strength-to-weight ratio, muscular endurance, and joint integrity you'll need in real-world scenarios.

This section focuses on bodyweight and minimal-equipment upper body training — scalable from beginner to advanced.

1. Push-Up (Standard and Variations)

Purpose:
Core upper body movement. Builds strength in the chest, shoulders, triceps, and core while reinforcing shoulder stability and body control.

Execution (Standard Push-Up):

1. Hands under shoulders or slightly wider.
2. Body in a straight line — head to heels.
3. Lower under control, chest to within a few centimeters of the ground.
4. Press back up — don't let hips sag or pike.

Common Mistakes:

- Flaring elbows too wide
- Sagging lower back
- Incomplete range (only half-reps)

Progressions:

- Diamond push-ups
- Tempo push-ups (3 sec down, 1 sec pause, 1 sec up)
- Ruck push-ups (load on back)

Regressions:

- Knee push-ups
- Incline push-ups (hands on bench or table)
- Reduced reps per set (focus on quality)

2. Pull-Up / Chin-Up

Purpose:
Critical for vertical pulling strength — used for climbing, vaulting, and scaling. One of the best indicators of relative upper body strength.

Execution (Standard Pull-Up):

1. Grip the bar, palms facing away (chin-up = palms toward you).
2. Start from full hang.
3. Pull chin above the bar with control.

4. Lower all the way down — full range every rep.

Common Mistakes:
- Half-reps (not lowering fully)
- Kipping or swinging
- Shrugged shoulders at start

Progressions:
- Weighted pull-ups
- Slow negatives (3–5 sec down)
- L-sit pull-ups (core + grip)

Regressions:
- Jumping pull-ups with slow negative
- Resistance band assisted pull-ups
- Inverted rows under a sturdy table/bar

3. Dips (Parallel Bars or Between Chairs)

Purpose:
Targets chest, triceps, and shoulders. Excellent for building pressing strength and shoulder mobility.

Execution:
1. Support yourself on parallel bars (or two chairs).
2. Lower slowly — elbows to 90° or deeper.
3. Press back up fully.

Common Mistakes:
- Shoulders rolling forward
- Shallow range
- Flaring elbows

Progressions:
- Weighted dips

- Slow eccentric (lowering)
- Ring dips (adds instability)

Regressions:

- Bench dips (feet on floor)
- Leg-supported dips
- Partial range

4. Inverted Rows

Purpose:
Builds upper back, arms, and grip. Easier than pull-ups but still excellent for strength and posture.

Execution:

1. Use a low bar or table.
2. Grip bar, keep body straight.
3. Pull chest to bar, squeeze shoulder blades.
4. Lower slowly and repeat.

Common Mistakes:

- Hips sagging
- Not pulling fully
- Using momentum

Progressions:

- Feet elevated
- Weighted vest
- Tempo rows

Regressions:

- Bend knees
- Reduce reps
- Increase rest between sets

5. Pike Push-Up / Shoulder Press Progression

Purpose:
Develops shoulder strength for vertical pressing, mimicking overhead work in confined spaces or when gear limits motion.

Execution (Pike Push-Up):

1. Start in downward dog position — hips high, arms straight.
2. Lower head toward the floor between hands.
3. Press back up with control.

Common Mistakes:

- Not keeping elbows close
- Arching lower back
- Moving in a straight line instead of diagonal

Progressions:

- Elevated feet pike push-up
- Handstand push-up (against wall)
- Wall walk + shoulder tap holds

Regressions:

- Decrease range of motion
- Knee pike push-up
- Wall shoulder presses with light weight

6. Wall Climb / Climbing Prep

Purpose:
Builds scapular control, grip endurance, and confidence for climbing obstacles, fences, and ropes.

Execution (Wall Climb):

1. Start in plank position with feet against a wall.
2. Slowly walk feet up the wall while hands move closer.
3. Pause at 45° or go vertical (handstand).

4. Reverse slowly to return.

Common Mistakes:

- Rushing
- Losing tension in midline
- Going beyond control level

Progressions:

- Full handstand hold
- Wall walks to handstand push-up
- Combine with shoulder taps

Regressions:

- Partial wall climb (45° only)
- Feet on box for elevation
- Isometric holds mid-range

Lower Body Movements

Lower body strength isn't just about powerful legs — it's about building a foundation that can carry weight, absorb impact, and move with purpose under stress. In tactical environments, your legs are your engine. Whether you're sprinting to cover, climbing hills with a ruck, or holding a defensive position, you need durability, balance, and endurance from the ground up.

This section breaks down the most essential lower-body movements, scaled from beginner to advanced, using just your bodyweight or minimal gear.

1. Air Squat (Bodyweight Squat)

Purpose:
Builds foundational strength in the quads, glutes, hamstrings, and core. Reinforces proper movement mechanics and balance.

Execution:

1. Stand with feet shoulder-width apart.

2. Lower hips back and down — knees track over toes, chest stays tall.

3. Go as deep as mobility allows (preferably below parallel).

4. Drive through heels to return to standing.

Common Mistakes:

- Knees caving in

- Heels lifting off the ground

- Rounding the back

Progressions:

- Jump squats

- Tempo squats (3–1–1 tempo)

- Ruck squats (add weight via backpack)

Regressions:

- Box squats (sit back onto a box or bench)

- Shallow range

- Use a wall for support

2. Split Squat / Bulgarian Split Squat

Purpose:
Improves unilateral strength, balance, and stability. Addresses muscle imbalances between legs and reinforces hip mobility.

Execution:

1. Stand in a split stance. Rear foot elevated on a bench or step (Bulgarian style).

2. Lower back knee toward the ground with control.

3. Front knee should not push far past toes.

4. Drive through the front heel to return to standing.

Common Mistakes:

- Wobbling knees
- Leaning too far forward
- Poor depth control

Progressions:

- Weighted split squats (dumbbells or ruck)
- Pause at bottom
- Explosive drive (jump switch)

Regressions:

- Bodyweight only
- Rear foot on ground (regular split squat)
- Shorter range of motion

3. Step-Up

Purpose:
Practical movement for climbing, hiking, and loading the legs independently. Excellent for knee health and strength under load.

Execution:

1. Use a box, bench, or step (knee-height or slightly lower).
2. Step up with control — drive through the top leg only.
3. Stand fully upright.
4. Step down carefully, keeping tension.

Common Mistakes:

- Pushing off the trailing leg
- Not standing fully
- Losing balance on descent

Progressions:

- Ruck-loaded step-ups

- Step-up to knee drive (balance challenge)
- Slow eccentric descent

Regressions:

- Lower height
- Hold a wall for support
- Fewer reps per leg

4. Lunge (Forward, Reverse, Walking)

Purpose:
Builds dynamic leg strength, balance, and hip stability. Lunges also prepare you for changing direction quickly — vital in field settings.

Execution:

1. Step forward (or backward) with one leg.
2. Lower until both knees are at ~90°.
3. Keep torso upright, weight centered.
4. Drive back to start or step through.

Common Mistakes:

- Front knee collapsing inward
- Leaning the torso forward
- Shallow depth

Progressions:

- Walking lunges with a ruck
- Jumping lunges
- Pause lunges (1–2 second hold at the bottom)

Regressions:

- Static lunge in place
- Shortened range
- Hold onto the wall or rail

5. Glute Bridge / Hip Thrust

Purpose:
Builds posterior chain strength — glutes, hamstrings, and core. Crucial for sprinting, rucking, and preventing lower back strain.

Execution (Glute Bridge):
1. Lie on your back, knees bent, feet flat.
2. Press through heels to lift hips.
3. Squeeze glutes at the top.
4. Lower under control.

Common Mistakes:
- Hyperextending the lower back
- Pushing through toes
- Not activating glutes (letting hamstrings take over)

Progressions:
- Single-leg glute bridge
- Ruck-loaded hip thrust
- Elevated feet

Regressions:
- Shorter range
- Use both feet closer to the glutes
- Reduce reps, increase rest

6. Jump Squat / Bounding

Purpose:
Develops power, explosiveness, and coordination. Trains your ability to generate force quickly — key in tactical movement.

Execution:
1. Start in a bodyweight squat.
2. Explode up into a jump, fully extending hips and knees.

3. Land softly with knees slightly bent, back into a squat.

4. Reset and repeat.

Common Mistakes:
- Stiff, hard landings
- Collapsing knees on landing
- Using arms excessively (flailing)

Progressions:
- Tuck jumps
- Broad jumps
- Ruck jump squats (advanced only)

Regressions:
- Low bounce (barely leave the ground)
- Remove jump — explosive stand only
- Fewer reps, more rest

7. Ruck March / Loaded Carry

Purpose:
Simulates field conditioning — carrying weight over distance. Builds leg endurance, traps, grip, and posture under fatigue.

Execution:
1. Use a backpack (10–20 kg depending on level).
2. Walk at a steady pace (20–60 minutes).
3. Maintain upright posture, don't hunch.
4. Focus on efficient foot strike and breathing.

Common Mistakes:
- Slouching under load
- Taking oversized steps
- Not hydrating before/after

Progressions:

- Increase weight or distance
- Add terrain (hills, trails)
- Timed marches (e.g., 5 km under 45 minutes)

Regressions:

- Lighter ruck
- Shorter time (10–20 min)

12. Stay Mission-Ready: Life After the 6 Weeks

You've completed the 6-week tactical training plan. You've moved with discipline, trained with purpose, and fueled your body like a soldier. But now comes the real challenge: what's next?

Fitness isn't just a phase. If you want lasting results — strength, endurance, mental toughness — you need to treat this like a long-term mission. This chapter is about keeping your edge, evolving your training, and staying mission-ready without burning out or falling off track. Because tactical readiness doesn't end. It adapts.

Redefine the Mission

The biggest mistake people make after completing a program is returning to old habits — no plan, no structure, no accountability. Don't let that be you.

Your mission doesn't end at week six. It changes form.

Now, instead of following a fixed plan, your mission becomes:

- Maintain and build on your fitness base
- Set new challenges aligned with your goals
- Stay consistent without rigid burnout
- Train smart to avoid injury and overtraining

Start by redefining your objective. Ask:

- Do I want to improve my endurance now?

- Do I want to get stronger and increase reps?

- Do I want to focus on body composition and fat loss?

- Do I want to prepare for a specific event (military test, ruck march, obstacle course)?

Pick one primary goal for the next 6 to 12 weeks. Keep your purpose clear, or you'll drift.

Create Your Ongoing Training Framework

Let's break down a sustainable tactical training structure you can repeat, adapt, and evolve.

Weekly Template (Baseline Maintenance Phase)

Day 1 – Full Body Strength + Core
Day 2 – Conditioning (Intervals or Circuits) + Mobility
Day 3 – Strength Focus (Upper or Lower) + Core
Day 4 – Active Recovery or Mobility
Day 5 – Long Cardio or Tactical Endurance (e.g., ruck march)
Day 6 – Full Body Circuit + Core
Day 7 – Rest or Light Walk/Yoga

You don't need to follow this rigidly. Think of it as a mission protocol you can modify based on time, stress, or recovery. The idea is to hit all the key systems every week:

- Strength (2–3x)

- Conditioning (1–2x)

- Core (3x)

- Endurance (1x)

- Mobility (2–3x)

- Recovery (1–2x)

If you're tight on time, reduce volume — not frequency. A 20-minute focused session is better than skipping entirely.

Progressive Overload Doesn't Stop

The human body adapts fast. What pushed you in Week 1 of the program might feel easy now. That's not a sign to relax — it's a sign to level up.

Ways to apply progressive overload after the 6-week plan:

- Increase reps (e.g., from 30 to 40 push-ups)
- Decrease rest time (e.g., 60 sec → 30 sec between rounds)
- Add weight (ruck, backpack, sandbag)
- Add rounds to circuits
- Introduce harder variations (e.g., dive bomber push-ups, jumping lunges)

Your goal is simple: keep the body guessing. When you feel comfortable, it's time to change something.

Mix Tactical and Personal Goals

The best way to stay engaged is to set new personal benchmarks.

Examples:

- Complete a 2-mile run in under 14 minutes
- Perform 20 strict pull-ups
- Hold a 3-minute plank
- Complete 10 rounds of a specific circuit without stopping
- Pass the Army Combat Fitness Test (ACFT) or Marine PFT

Tactical training isn't just about surviving workouts. It's about becoming a more capable human being.

Mission-Specific Tracks

Depending on your next goal, you may want to follow a more specialized training path. Here's how to shift focus while keeping tactical readiness intact.

➤ Strength Focus

- Prioritize progressive bodyweight work (push-ups, pull-ups, squats)
- Add loaded carries (farmer walks, ruck carries)
- Track reps over time
- Train lower rep ranges (5–10) with more difficulty
- Focus on controlled tempo and time under tension

➤ Fat Loss Focus

- Increase circuit and HIIT-style sessions (3–4x/week)
- Add fasted morning walks or light cardio
- Keep strength 2x/week to preserve muscle
- Monitor caloric intake and protein

➤ Endurance Focus

- Add weekly long runs or rucks (build up to 60–90 mins)
- Use heart rate zones or RPE to pace
- Include intervals to improve VO2 max
- Fuel appropriately before long sessions

Switch tracks every 6–8 weeks, or when progress plateaus.

Deload Weeks: Built-In Recovery

Burnout is real. Especially if you're pushing hard, tracking progress, and stacking reps every week.

Every 6–8 weeks, plan a deload week:

- Cut workout volume by 40–50%

- Reduce training intensity (no PRs or max reps)

- Focus on recovery: sleep, food, hydration, walking, mobility

- Reflect on goals and reset your plan

Think of it as maintenance on your equipment. You're not being lazy — you're extending your mission capability.

Use Technology and Tracking Tools

Stay accountable and motivated by tracking progress.

Tools to consider:

- Training journal (appendix or digital)

- Spreadsheet for reps, times, and weights

- Apps like Strong, MyFitnessPal, or Strava

- Fitness watch to monitor heart rate zones and steps

Write down your numbers. Don't rely on memory. The data tells the story of your discipline.

Recovery Is Still Part of the Plan

Don't confuse "training" with always going hard.

Tactical readiness requires balance:

- **Sleep** – Aim for 7–9 hours/night. It's your #1 recovery tool.

- **Mobility** – Don't skip it. Tight muscles lead to poor form and injury.

- **Nutrition** – Keep fueling based on your current mission.

- **Stress Management** – Walk, breathe, take rest days. Your nervous system needs decompression.

Recovery isn't weakness. It's strategic regeneration.

Tactical Fitness = Lifelong Readiness

The 6-week plan got you moving, sweating, and progressing. But the real reward is in making this part of your lifestyle.

You don't need a new program every month. You need consistency. You need a challenge. You need discipline.

Remember:

- You've already built the foundation
- You have the tools to self-program
- You've proven you can follow through

You're now in a position most people never reach — you've trained with a soldier's mindset and results-driven system. Now it's time to own that.

Examples of Long-Term Weekly Training Splits

To help you visualize how to maintain and progress over the next 3–6 months, here are two adaptable templates:

Example 1 – Balanced Maintenance (Strength + Conditioning)

Day Focus

Mon Full Body Strength + Core

Tue Conditioning (Intervals)

Wed Upper Body Strength + Mobility

Thu Ruck or Run (Endurance)

Fri Full Body Circuit

Sat Optional: Light Cardio or Skill Work

Sun Rest or Active Recovery

Example 2 – Strength & Muscle Focus

Day Focus

Mon Upper Body Strength

Day Focus

Tue   Conditioning + Core

Wed Lower Body Strength

Thu   Recovery & Mobility

Fri   Tactical Circuit

Sat   Ruck or Weighted Sled

Sun Rest

You Are Your Own Commander Now

You've made it through the full tactical plan. You've learned how to show up, work hard, fuel with discipline, and recover with intention. Now, the responsibility — and the reward — is in your hands.

You don't need a drill instructor to keep you going. You've built the mindset to do that on your own.

Stay sharp.

Keep evolving.

And remember: the mission never ends, it just levels up.

13. Bonus Content & Resources

This chapter is your field manual for ongoing support. You've completed the core program, but the mission doesn't end here. Use this section as your personal resource center for tracking, adapting, and continuing your tactical journey.

We've included the following:

1. **Training Logs & Templates**
2. **Assessment Tracker (Day 0 / Week 6 / Long-Term)**
3. **Progression Variations for Bodyweight Movements**
4. **Tactical Gear Guide (Minimal Equipment)**
5. **Suggested Reading & Learning Resources**

Let's break each of these down.

1. Training Logs & Templates

Tracking your workouts is critical for long-term success. If you're not measuring your performance, you're guessing. Use these templates to log your reps, time, effort, and weekly wins.

Daily Training Log (Example):

Date	Workout Name	Sets/Reps	Notes
9/14	Conditioning Circuit A	3 rounds – 20 push-ups, 30 squats, 15 burpees	Felt strong – decreased rest time
9/16	Run	2 miles in 17:45	HR stayed under 160, a big improvement

Print or copy these for daily use, or plug them into a notes app or spreadsheet.

Weekly Check-In (Every 7 Days):

- ☑ Did I complete all workouts?

- ✅ Did I eat to support my training?

- ✅ How do I feel physically? (1–10 scale)

- ✅ How do I feel mentally?

- ✅ 1 thing I did well:

- ✅ 1 thing I'll improve next week:

Build a habit of self-assessment. Stay accountable.

2. Assessment Tracker

You already performed baseline assessments in Chapter 4. Use this format to track both short-term and long-term progress. Record Day 0, Week 6, and any checkpoint after.

Test	Day 0	Week 6	3-Month
Max Push-ups (2 min)	28	42	—
Max Planck Hold	1:10	2:15	—
1.5-Mile Run	14:40	13:05	—
Squats in 1 min	45	58	—
Pull-ups	3	6	—
Mobility Test (pass/fail)	Fail	Pass	—

Don't aim for perfection — aim for measurable improvement.

3. Bodyweight Progressions

To keep improving without needing a gym, here's a list of key movements and how to increase difficulty over time.

Push-up Progressions:

- Incline push-ups → Standard push-ups → Diamond push-ups → Archer push-ups → Feet-elevated push-ups → Clap push-ups

Pull-up Progressions:

- Negative reps → Band-assisted → Strict → Weighted → L-sit → Archer or towel variations

Squat Progressions:

- Air squats → Pause squats → Jump squats → Bulgarian split squats → Pistol squats → Weighted squats (ruck or sandbag)

Core:

- Dead bug → Hollow hold → Plank → Plank with reach → L-sit → Hanging leg raises

Don't try to jump levels overnight. Master the basics, then layer difficulty slowly.

4. Minimal Tactical Gear Guide

You don't need much to train like a soldier — but here are tools that expand your options, especially for home or field training.

Item	Use
Pull-up Bar (doorframe or outdoor)	Essential for back and arm strength
Ruck or Backpack (10–30kg)	Weighted marches, squats, push-ups
Sandbag or Kettlebell	Carries, cleans, overhead press
Jump Rope	Conditioning + footwork
Resistance Bands	Warm-up, mobility, and assisted pull-ups

Item	Use
Timer App or Interval Timer	For circuits, intervals, and recovery tracking

Use gear as a multiplier — not a crutch. If you ever lose access, you should still be able to train.

5. Suggested Reading & Resources

Continue building your mindset and knowledge base. Here are highly recommended resources.

Training & Performance:

- *Built to Endure* – by Cameron Hanes
- *The Naked Warrior* – by Pavel Tsatsouline
- *You Can't Hurt Me* – by David Goggins
- *Becoming a Supple Leopard* – by Dr. Kelly Starrett

Nutrition:

- *The Renaissance Diet 2.0* – Dr. Mike Israetel
- *The Performance Nutrition Handbook* – Precision Nutrition
- *The Warfighter Nutrition Guide* – U.S. Army (free PDF online)

Military Fitness Standards (U.S.):

- Army Combat Fitness Test (ACFT)
- Marine Corps Physical Fitness Test (PFT)
- Navy Physical Readiness Test (PRT)

Mobility & Recovery:

- *The Ready State* App (Dr. Kelly Starrett)
- *GOWOD* (great for daily mobility)
- *Yoga for Veterans* (free routines on YouTube)

Final Mission Reminder

You've reached the end of the book — but not the end of the work. This resource section is here for you whenever you need to reset, reframe, or rebuild.

Whether you're starting over, leveling up, or preparing for a new challenge, the foundation is always the same:

- Discipline
- Consistency
- Simplicity
- Execution

Use this chapter to fuel your independence. You are now your own coach, your own commander, and your own motivator. Never forget to always believe in yourself, and even when everything turns dark, look for your inner light. I believe in you.

www.ingramcontent.com/pod-product-compliance
Lightning Source LLC
Chambersburg PA
CBHW061042110426
42740CB00050B/2845